COMPLETE GUIDE TO UNDERSTANDING CORONARY ARTERY BYPASS GRAFTING

Essential Resource On Procedures, Post-Operative Care, Heart Health, Recovery, Risks, And Patient Care

KLEIN HOYLE

Disclaimer

The content in this book is based on the author's expertise and comprehension of the topic. The author has no affiliation or link with any corporation, business, or person. This book is meant to give general information and educational material only, and it should not be interpreted as professional medical advice. Always seek the advice of a skilled healthcare expert if you have any queries about medical issues or treatments. The author and publisher expressly disclaim any responsibility resulting directly or indirectly from the use or use of the information included in this book.

Table of Contents

ABOUT THIS BOOK

The "Complete Guide to Understanding Coronary Artery Bypass Grafting" is an invaluable resource for medical professionals, patients, and anybody seeking in-depth information regarding CABG. Since its debut, CABG has been a cornerstone in the treatment of coronary artery disease, providing patients with a route to better heart health and quality of life. This book not only explains the historical history and purpose of CABG but also goes into the detailed architecture of the heart and coronary arteries, revealing their critical function in cardiovascular health.

One of This book's notable aspects is its thorough examination of the indications for CABG. By presenting the symptoms, diagnostic tests, and patient profiles that necessitate CABG consideration, readers get a comprehensive knowledge of when this treatment is the best course of action. Furthermore, the full explanation of preoperative preparations emphasizes the significance of complete patient care, which includes consultations, assessments, and psychological support.

This book's heart resides in its extensive description of the CABG operation. Readers learn about the complexities of this life-saving procedure by delving into surgical methods, surgical team duties, and postoperative care standards. Furthermore, This book discusses possible risks and consequences connected with CABG, equipping both patients and healthcare practitioners to manage these issues through proactive steps and diligent monitoring.

Beyond the initial surgical phase, This book discusses long-term treatment and lifestyle changes. It promotes a comprehensive approach to heart health by providing food advice, exercise guidelines, and drug management tips. Furthermore, investigating improvements and alternatives in CABG sheds light on the ever-changing environment of cardiovascular surgery, offering a look into future trends and developments that promise to improve patient outcomes even further.

In short, the "Complete Guide to Understanding Coronary Artery Bypass Grafting" is more than just an instructional guidebook; it is a source of information, compassion, and hope for anyone navigating the difficulties of coronary artery disease and cardiac surgery. Whether you're a healthcare professional looking to expand your knowledge or a patient beginning on the CABG adventure, this book will serve as a valued companion, guiding you with clarity and expertise every step of the way.

CHAPTER 1

Introduction To Coronary Artery Bypass Grafting (CABG)

Definition And Purpose Of CABG

Coronary Artery Bypass Grafting (CABG) is a surgical treatment that increases blood flow to the heart. It entails removing a blood vessel from another region of the body and grafting it to bypass a blocked or restricted coronary artery. This new channel permits blood to flow around the obstruction, ensuring that the heart muscle gets enough oxygen and nutrients. CABG is generally used to treat coronary artery disease (CAD), a disorder marked by the accumulation of plaque in the coronary arteries, which may cause chest discomfort (angina), heart attacks, and other significant cardiovascular issues.

CABG serves several purposes, including relieving symptoms such as chest discomfort, improving the patient's quality of life, improving heart function, and lowering the risk of heart attack. For many patients with severe CAD, CABG may be a life-saving operation, significantly increasing life expectancy and general health.

History And Development Of The Procedure

CABG stretches back to the mid-twentieth century, with considerable developments happening throughout the years. The first successful coronary artery bypass surgery was done in the 1960s by Dr. René Favaloro, an Argentine cardiovascular surgeon. He pioneered a procedure that became standard practice in cardiac surgery by bypassing the blocked coronary artery using a piece of the patient's saphenous vein from the leg.

The process has been improved multiple times throughout the years. Early advancements included the use of the internal mammary artery as a graft, which has been found to provide greater long-term patency than vein grafts. Technological improvements, such as the creation of heart-lung machines, have also contributed significantly to the progress of CABG, enabling surgeons to operate on a still heart while preserving circulation and oxygen.

In the 1990s, minimally invasive procedures and off-pump operations were launched, which reduced the necessity for major incisions and the utilization of a heart-lung machine. These developments have resulted in faster recovery periods, fewer problems, and better results for patients.

The Importance Of CABG In Treating Coronary Artery Disease

CABG is an important intervention in the treatment of coronary artery disease, particularly for patients who have numerous blocked arteries, and severe angina or have not reacted well to alternative therapies such as medication or percutaneous coronary interventions (PCI). The technique has the potential to considerably reduce angina symptoms, minimize the need for anti-anginal drugs, and enhance exercise tolerance, thus improving patients' overall quality of life.

In addition to symptom alleviation, CABG has been demonstrated to increase survival rates in some patient groups, notably those with left main coronary artery disease, multiple vascular disease, and decreased left ventricular function. CABG decreases the risk of future heart attacks by restoring enough blood flow to the heart muscle.

The significance of CABG goes beyond individual patient outcomes. It also has a substantial influence on public health, since coronary artery disease is still one of the top causes of mortality globally. By efficiently treating severe instances of CAD, CABG helps to reduce the cardiovascular disease burden on healthcare systems and society as a whole.

CHAPTER 2

Anatomy Of The Heart And Coronary Arteries

Basic Structure And Function Of The Heart

The heart is a muscular organ about the size of a fist that sits slightly to the left of the middle of the chest. It has four chambers: two atria (upper chambers) and two ventricles (bottom chambers). The right atrium takes deoxygenated blood from the body via the superior and inferior vena cava and pumps it to the right ventricle. The right ventricle then circulates this blood to the lungs via the pulmonary artery for oxygenation.

Once oxygenated, the blood flows back to the left atrium via the pulmonary veins. The left atrium pumps oxygen-rich blood to the left ventricle, which then transports it to the rest of the body via the aorta, the body's biggest artery. The sinoatrial (SA) node, the heart's natural pacemaker, generates electrical impulses that cause rhythmic contractions.

The heart's walls are made up of three layers: epicardium (outer layer), myocardium (middle muscular layer), and endocardium (inner layer). The myocardium is very important because it allows the heart to pump blood effectively. The heart also has valves (tricuspid, pulmonary, mitral, and aortic) that maintain unidirectional blood flow and avoid backflow during contractions.

Coronary Arteries: Their Role In Heart Health

The coronary arteries are crucial blood vessels that carry oxygenated blood and nutrients to the heart muscle (myocardium), ensuring its proper function and survival.

The two major coronary arteries are the left coronary artery (LCA) and the right coronary artery (RCA).

The LCA is further divided into two arteries: the left anterior descending (LAD) and the circumflex (LCx). The LAD sends blood to the front and bottom of the left ventricle, as well as the septum, while the LCx gives blood to the left atrium, side, and rear of the left ventricle. The RCA pumps blood to the right atrium, right ventricle, and parts of the left ventricle and septum.

The coronary arteries start in the aorta, just above the aortic valve. Given the heart's constant and demanding strain, any reduction in coronary blood flow might cause serious health problems. Adequate coronary circulation is critical for the myocardium's function and overall heart health.

Common Coronary Artery Issues

Several disorders may limit the coronary arteries' capacity to provide enough blood to the heart muscle. Some of the most typical difficulties are:

1. Atherosclerosis is the accumulation of plaque (fat, cholesterol, and other chemicals) on the inner walls of the arteries. Over time, this plaque hardens and narrows the arteries, reducing blood flow.

2. **Coronary Artery Spasm:** This is a transient contraction of the muscles inside the artery walls that may decrease or stop blood flow to the heart. Although spasms are normally transient, they might induce chest discomfort (angina).

3. Coronary Artery Disease (CAD) is a wide term that refers to a variety of disorders that decrease blood flow through the coronary arteries owing to atherosclerosis or other causes. It is the major cause of heart attacks.

4. Coronary Artery Anomalies: Some people are born with atypical coronary artery architecture, which may lead to poor blood flow and cardiac issues.

5. Coronary Microvascular Disease (MVD) damages the heart's small arteries and may induce chest discomfort (angina) in the absence of visible blockages in the bigger coronary arteries.

How Coronary Artery Disease Develops

Coronary artery disease (CAD) progresses over time owing to a mix of hereditary, lifestyle, and environmental influences. The process often starts with damage or injury to the inner layer of a coronary artery. Several factors may contribute to this damage, including smoking, high blood pressure, high cholesterol, diabetes, and inflammation.

Atherosclerosis may develop when the inner lining of an artery is damaged. Low-density lipoprotein (LDL) cholesterol, sometimes known as "bad" cholesterol, accumulates in arterial walls, producing plaques. As these plaques accumulate, they may restrict the arteries and reduce blood flow to the heart muscle.

Inflammation also contributes significantly to the development of CAD. The body's immune system treats the cholesterol deposits as if they were injuries, sending white blood cells to engulf LDL cholesterol. This procedure increases inflammation, which may further constrict the artery.

Plaques may rupture over time, resulting in the formation of a blood clot on their surface. If a blood clot is big enough, it may stop the flow of blood via the coronary artery, causing a heart attack. Even partial blockages may create serious issues, such as angina (chest discomfort) during physical activity or stress.

Regular risk factor monitoring, a healthy lifestyle, and medical treatments are critical for CAD management and prevention.

CHAPTER 3
Indications For CABG

Symptoms That May Prompt CABG Consideration

Coronary Artery Bypass Grafting (CABG) is often explored when a patient exhibits symptoms of severe coronary artery disease (CAD) that cannot be properly treated with medicines or less invasive treatments. These symptoms usually include chest discomfort or angina, which may occur during physical activity or rest. Angina is often characterized as a sensation of pressure, squeezing, heaviness, or tightness in the chest, which might spread to the arms, shoulders, neck, jaw, or back.

Patients may also have shortness of breath, known as dyspnea, particularly after exercise or when resting flat.

This happens because the heart muscle may not be getting enough oxygen-rich blood to satisfy its demands, resulting in decreased cardiac performance. Fatigue and weakness are other frequent symptoms as the heart strains to efficiently pump blood throughout the body.

In certain situations, patients may exhibit signs of heart failure, such as edema in the legs, ankles, or feet, as well as trouble completing everyday tasks owing to diminished cardiac output. These symptoms suggest severe coronary artery disease, which may warrant CABG to increase blood flow to the heart muscle and reduce discomfort.

Diagnostic Testing And Assessments

Before deciding if a patient is a candidate for CABG, numerous diagnostic tests and assessments are usually performed to examine the amount of coronary artery disease and the general health of the heart. These tests may include:

1. Electrocardiogram (ECG/EKG): This test measures the electrical activity of the heart and may identify irregular rhythms, ischemia (insufficient oxygen to the heart muscle), and past heart attacks.

2. Echocardiogram: An echocardiogram employs sound waves to generate pictures of the heart's structure and function, enabling clinicians to evaluate the heart's pumping function and diagnose anomalies in the heart valves or chambers.

3. Stress testing consists of exercising on a treadmill or stationary cycle while measuring heart rate, blood pressure, and symptoms. This test assesses how effectively the heart reacts to increasing strain and may detect regions with decreased blood supply to the heart muscle.

4. Coronary angiography: This invasive treatment includes injecting a contrast dye into the coronary arteries and obtaining X-ray pictures (angiograms) to detect any blockages or narrowing. It offers extensive information on the location and degree of coronary artery disease.

5. Cardiac catheterization: This process involves inserting a thin, flexible tube (catheter) into a blood artery in the groin or arm and threading it to the coronary arteries. A contrast dye is then injected to help view the arteries and monitor blood pressure inside the heart chambers.

Conditions That Justify CABG Over Alternative Therapies

While CABG is a very efficient therapy for coronary artery disease, it is not usually the first choice and may only be used for individuals with certain diseases or features. CABG may be considered above alternative therapies in the following cases:

1. Severe coronary artery disease: Patients with significant blockages in numerous coronary arteries or left main coronary artery disease may benefit more from CABG than percutaneous coronary intervention (PCI) with stenting because CABG allows for more thorough revascularization.

2. Diabetes: Patients with diabetes and coronary artery disease often have more diffuse and complicated lesions, which may be treated more effectively with CABG than PCI. CABG has been demonstrated to have better long-term results in diabetes individuals than PCI.

3. Reduced heart function: Patients with severe left ventricular dysfunction or heart failure may benefit from CABG because revascularization may improve cardiac function and relieve symptoms.

4. Anatomical considerations: CABG may be preferable in patients with anatomical aspects that make PCI technically difficult, such as severely calcified or convoluted veins, or lesions at bifurcations or trifurcations.

Risk Factors And Patient Characteristics

When choosing CABG, it is critical to evaluate the patient's overall risk profile and the possibility of benefit from the treatment. Several variables might impact the choice to continue with CABG, including:

1. **Age:** Because advanced age is linked with higher surgical risk, older patients should be carefully assessed to see if the possible advantages of CABG exceed the hazards.

2. **Comorbidities:** Patients with other medical problems, such as hypertension, diabetes, renal disease, or lung illness, may be more likely to have difficulties during surgery and may need further preoperative optimization.

3. Smoking increases the risk of coronary artery disease and may hurt surgical results. Patients who smoke are advised to quit before receiving CABG to lessen the risk of postoperative problems.

4. Obesity: Obesity increases the risk of surgical complications and may have an impact on long-term results after CABG. Weight control methods may be advised before surgery to improve results.

5. Past cardiac history: Patients who have had past heart attacks, coronary artery bypass surgery, or PCI may have more complicated coronary artery disease and may need multiple CABG operations.

By carefully examining these risk variables and patient profiles, healthcare practitioners may make educated judgments regarding whether CABG is suitable for particular patients and improve post-operative outcomes.

CHAPTER 4

Preparing For CABG Surgery

Pre-Operative Consultations And Assessments

Before having coronary artery bypass grafting (CABG) surgery, you will have multiple consultations and examinations to ensure that you are both physically and psychologically prepared. These meetings are critical stages in the preoperative procedure, enabling your healthcare team to learn about your medical history, current health state, and any possible risks related to the operation.

During these consultations, you will meet with members of your healthcare team, such as your heart surgeon, cardiologist, anesthesiologist, and other medical specialists. They will undertake a full examination of your cardiovascular health, including electrocardiograms (ECGs), echocardiograms, and angiograms, to evaluate your heart's condition and establish the amount of coronary artery disease (CAD).

Your medical team will also go over your medical history, including any pre-existing diseases, prior surgeries, allergies, and drugs you are presently taking. It is critical to offer precise and complete information during these consultations to guarantee your safety throughout the operation and recuperation period.

Your healthcare team will create a customized treatment plan based on the outcomes of these examinations, taking into account your individual requirements and medical condition. This plan will define the suggested course of action, such as the kind of CABG operation, the quantity of grafts required, and any other therapies or interventions that may be necessary.

In addition to assessing your physical health, your healthcare team will analyze your emotional and psychological well-being to ensure that you are emotionally prepared for surgery and the difficulties of recovery. They will give information and assistance to reduce any anxieties or concerns you may have, as well as answer any questions or doubts you may have concerning the treatment.

General, pre-surgical consultations and assessments are crucial phases in the CABG surgery preparation process, enabling your healthcare team to collect vital information, evaluate your general health, and create a complete treatment plan suited to your requirements and circumstances.

Medications And Lifestyle Modifications Before Surgery

In preparation for CABG surgery, your healthcare team may prescribe certain drugs and lifestyle modifications to improve your health and lower the risk of problems during and after the treatment. These therapies are intended to improve your cardiovascular health, stabilize your condition, and improve the result of the procedure.

Aspirin, one of the most often recommended drugs before CABG surgery, helps prevent blood clots and lowers the risk of heart attack and stroke. To further lower the chance of clot formation, your doctor may prescribe additional blood thinners such as clopidogrel or warfarin.

In addition to drugs, your healthcare provider may recommend lifestyle modifications to enhance your general health and well-being. This might involve stopping smoking, eating a balanced diet low in saturated fats and cholesterol, increasing physical exercise, and reducing stress.

Quitting smoking is especially crucial before CABG surgery since it dramatically increases the risk of problems including infection, poor wound healing, and cardiovascular events. Your healthcare team can provide you with information and assistance to help you stop smoking and overcome any nicotine addiction concerns.

A nutritious diet rich in fruits, vegetables, whole grains, and lean meats may help decrease cholesterol, lower blood pressure, and enhance overall heart health. Your doctor or dietitian can help you establish a heart-healthy eating plan that is personalized to your specific requirements and interests.

Regular physical exercise is also required to improve cardiovascular fitness, strengthen the heart muscle, and lower the risk of problems before and after a CABG operation. Your healthcare provider may offer exercise routines and activities that are suitable for your current fitness level and medical condition.

Stress management is another important component of preparation for CABG surgery, since it may worsen cardiovascular symptoms and raise the risk of complications. Deep breathing exercises, meditation, yoga, and mindfulness are all techniques that may help decrease stress while also promoting relaxation and well-being.

Overall, drugs and lifestyle adjustments before CABG surgery are critical for maximizing your health, lowering the risk of problems, and increasing the procedure's results. By following your healthcare team's advice and implementing positive lifestyle changes, you may improve your overall cardiovascular health and prepare for a successful surgery and recovery.

Hospital Admission And Preoperative Preparations

On the day of your CABG operation, you will be admitted to the hospital and given preoperative instructions to ensure that you are prepared for the procedure. Hospital admission is usually arranged several hours before the intended operation time to allow for essential testing, evaluations, and preparations.

When you arrive at the hospital, you will be met by the nursing staff and sent to the preoperative section, where you will change into a hospital gown and go through several preparatory procedures. These may involve monitoring your vital signs, collecting blood for laboratory testing, inserting an intravenous (IV) line to deliver fluids and drugs, and examining your medical history and prescriptions.

Your healthcare team will also do a last examination to confirm that you are physically and psychologically prepared for the operation and that there are no new developments or concerns that must be addressed before continuing. This may include checking your permission paperwork, clarifying any last-minute questions or concerns, and verifying the surgical procedure's specifics.

In addition to these preoperative preparations, your healthcare team will give you pre-surgery instructions and recommendations. To limit the risk of infection, you may need to fast before the surgery, avoid certain medicines, and adhere to strict cleanliness and skincare regimens.

Depending on your specific requirements and medical condition, you may undergo additional interventions or treatments before surgery. For example, if you have diabetes, your blood sugar levels may need to be closely checked and regulated before the treatment. Similarly, if you have high blood pressure or other cardiovascular risk factors, your healthcare provider may offer additional drugs or therapies to help you manage your condition.

Overall, hospital admission and preoperative preparations are critical elements in the preparation process for CABG surgery, ensuring that you are ready for the treatment and that all required procedures and measures are in place to maximize your safety and well-being.

Psychological Preparation And Assistance

Preparing for CABG surgery entails not only physical preparedness but also psychological preparation and assistance to help you deal with the emotional and mental obstacles of the process. Surgery, particularly one as major as CABG, may be stressful and anxiety-provoking, and it is critical to address these concerns to encourage a happy surgical experience and recovery.

Your healthcare team will give information and assistance to help you overcome any thoughts or concerns you may have regarding the operation and recovery process. They will explain the process, what to anticipate before, during, and after surgery, and address any questions or concerns you may have.

In addition to the assistance offered by your healthcare team, you may choose to seek further psychological help from a therapist, counselor, or support group. These tools may offer a secure and supportive setting in which to vent your emotions, exchange experiences with others who have experienced comparable treatments, and learn coping skills for stress and anxiety.

Family members and loved ones may also be quite helpful in offering emotional support and encouragement during the medical procedure. Having a solid support system in place may help lessen emotions of loneliness, fear, and worry while also providing comfort and reassurance during this difficult time.

It is important to talk freely and honestly with your healthcare staff and loved ones about your emotions, worries, and requirements before surgery and throughout the recovery period. By obtaining help and proactively treating any psychological concerns, you may improve your general well-being and resilience, as well as prepare for a favorable surgical result.

To summarize, psychological preparation and support are critical components of preparing for CABG surgery, assisting you in dealing with the emotional and mental obstacles of the treatment and fostering a happy surgical experience and recovery. You may handle the surgical process with confidence and resilience by obtaining help from your healthcare team, loved ones, and any other resources that are required.

CHAPTER 5

The CABG Procedure

Types Of CABG Procedures

Coronary Artery Bypass Grafting (CABG) may be done using a variety of procedures, each adapted to the patient's condition and requirements.

On-Pump CABG

On-pump CABG involves briefly stopping the heart and having a heart-lung machine flow blood throughout the body. Surgeons then exploit this window of opportunity to bypass the clogged coronary arteries with transplanted blood vessels (grafts), usually from the leg or chest. This approach enables precision transplant implantation and comprehensive coronary artery access.

Off-pump CABG, commonly known as beating heart surgery, is conducted while the heart is still beating. This approach removes the need for a heart-lung machine, possibly lowering the risk of problems from its usage. Surgeons stabilize the portion of the heart where the transplant will be placed, allowing for accurate graft placement without disrupting the heart's function completely.

Minimally Invasive CABG

Minimally invasive CABG includes making tiny incisions and accessing the heart with specialist devices. When compared to standard open-heart surgery, this technique has fewer complications, shorter recovery periods, and a lower risk of infection. It may not be appropriate for all people or kinds of coronary artery blockages.

Detailed Steps Of Surgery

Preoperative preparation

Before the procedure, the patient is prepared and sedated. The surgical team ensures that all required equipment is prepared, and the patient's vital signs are continuously checked.

Harvesting Grafts

Grafts are harvested from appropriate blood arteries, such as the internal mammary artery, radial artery, or saphenous vein. These grafts will be utilized to open up new channels for blood flow around the obstructed coronary arteries.

Graft Placement

After the grafts are produced, the surgeon gently joins them to the coronary arteries beyond the obstructions. This gets around the blocked locations, restoring blood flow to the heart muscle.

After finishing the graft placements, the surgical team controls the bleeding and closes the wounds with sutures or staples.

Role Of The Surgical Team

A cardiovascular surgeon

The cardiovascular surgeon directs the surgical team and executes the CABG surgery. They are well-trained in heart surgery procedures and supervise the whole procedure.

Anesthesiologist

The anesthesiologist provides anesthetic to keep the patient asleep and pain-free throughout the treatment. They also monitor the patient's vital signs and alter the anesthetic as required.

Perfusionist

During on-pump CABG surgeries, the perfusionist runs the heart-lung machine, which keeps the patient's blood flowing and oxygenated while the heart stops.

Surgical Assistants
Surgical assistants help the cardiovascular surgeon throughout the surgery. They may help with graft preparation, tissue manipulation, and other responsibilities as assigned by the surgeon.

Duration And Immediate Post-Operative Care

Surgery Duration

The length of a CABG operation varies according to the amount of grafts required and the intricacy of the patient's condition. On average, the procedure might last three to six hours.

Immediate postoperative care

Following surgery, the patient is sent to the intensive care unit (ICU) for careful monitoring. Medical personnel check vital signs, provide pain medicine, and make sure the patient is comfortable and stable.

Respiratory Support

Patients may need respiratory assistance, such as mechanical ventilation, to help them breathe until they can do so independently.

Mobilization and Rehabilitation

Early mobilization and physical therapy are critical components of postsurgical treatment. Patients are recommended to gradually resume their physical activity to enhance healing and avoid problems such as blood clots and pneumonia.

Medication Management

Patients are given drugs to treat pain, prevent infection, and regulate blood pressure and cholesterol levels. These drugs promote recovery and lower the risk of problems.

Follow-up Care

After being discharged from the hospital, patients continue to get follow-up treatment from their healthcare professionals. This might involve frequent check-ups, cardiac rehabilitation programs, and medication modifications as required.

CHAPTER 6

Post-Operative Care And Recovery

Initial Recovery In The ICU

Following coronary artery bypass grafting (CABG), patients are usually moved to the Intensive Care Unit (ICU) for initial recovery and strict monitoring. The intensive care unit (ICU) offers a controlled environment in which healthcare specialists may carefully monitor vital signs, handle any immediate postoperative issues, and assure the patient's stability before moving to a normal hospital room.

Patients in the ICU will be attached to a variety of monitors that will continually check their heart rate, blood pressure, oxygen levels, and other vital signs. Medications, fluids, and any required blood transfusions will be administered via intravenous lines. Patients may also get a urinary catheter to precisely measure urine output.

Close supervision in the ICU enables healthcare staff to respond quickly to any difficulties that may occur, such as bleeding, abnormal heart rhythms, or breathing problems. Patients may be given supplementary oxygen via a nasal cannula or face mask to help them breathe if necessary. In addition, pain management will be used to maintain the patient's comfort throughout this vital phase of recuperation.

The duration of stay in the ICU varies according to the particular patient's health and the complexity of the procedure. Patients are often admitted to the intensive care unit (ICU) for at least the first 24 to 48 hours after CABG surgery. During this period, healthcare staff will constantly monitor the patient's development and eventually move them to a normal hospital room once they are stable and no longer need intensive care.

Pain Management And Wound Care

Pain management is an important part of postoperative therapy after CABG surgery. Patients may have varied degrees of discomfort or pain at the incision sites and in the chest as a result of surgical trauma. Effective pain management not only improves patient comfort but also promotes speedier recovery and allows for greater engagement in rehabilitation activities.

To relieve pain and inflammation, physicians may prescribe opioids, nonsteroidal anti-inflammatory medications (NSAIDs), and acetaminophen. These drugs are given orally, intravenously, or via patient-controlled analgesia (PCA) pumps, which enable patients to self-administer pain treatment as required within acceptable limits.

In addition to pharmaceutical therapies, adequate wound care is essential for encouraging healing and avoiding infection at surgical incision sites.

Healthcare personnel will monitor the incisions for symptoms of infection, such as redness, swelling, warmth, or discharge. Sterile dressings may be used to protect the wounds and provide a clean healing environment.

Patients will be given information on how to care for their wounds at home, including how to wash, change bandages, and watch for any symptoms of problems. To reduce infection risk and ensure optimum wound healing, please follow these directions.

Physical Therapy And Rehabilitation

Physical therapy and rehabilitation are essential in the healing process after CABG surgery. These therapies attempt to improve patients' overall quality of life by restoring strength, flexibility, and mobility, as well as improving their cardiovascular fitness.

Patients will begin modest workouts and mobility activities soon after surgery, guided by a physical therapist.

Deep breathing exercises, coughing activities to cleanse the lungs, and modest range-of-motion exercises for the arms and legs are all possible options.

As the patient's health stabilizes, physical therapy will move to increasingly difficult exercises targeted at increasing strength, endurance, and functional skills. Walking, stationary bike riding, stair climbing, and strength training activities with bands or weights are all possible options.

Rehabilitation programs are customized to each patient's specific requirements and may continue as outpatient care after release from the hospital. The objective is to assist patients restore independence in everyday tasks, return to employment or leisure activities, and lower their risk of future cardiovascular events via lifestyle changes and regular exercise.

Monitoring For Complications

Complication monitoring is an important element of postoperative treatment after CABG surgery since it allows for the early detection and management of any possible difficulties. Common consequences include infection, bleeding, fluid buildup around the heart or lungs (pericardial or pleural effusion), pneumonia, blood clots, and cardiac arrhythmias.

Healthcare personnel will regularly monitor the patient's vital signs, such as heart rate, blood pressure, temperature, and oxygen saturation, for any indications of worsening or problems. Regular laboratory tests, such as blood counts, electrolyte levels, and cardiac enzymes, may be conducted to check organ function and discover anomalies.

Imaging tests, such as chest X-rays or echocardiograms, may be conducted to assess the heart and lungs and discover structural problems or fluid buildup.

These tests allow healthcare practitioners to make more informed judgments regarding the patient's treatment and management.

Early detection and management are critical in preventing problems from worsening and improving patient outcomes. Patients should notify their healthcare professionals as soon as they notice any new or worsening symptoms, such as chest discomfort, shortness of breath, fever, or edema, to ensure rapid examination and treatment. Healthcare practitioners may assist patients following CABG surgery to recover more smoothly by regularly monitoring for problems and offering appropriate therapies.

CHAPTER 7

Potential Risks And Complications

Common Risks Of CABG

Coronary Artery Bypass Grafting (CABG) is a significant surgical treatment that, like other surgeries, includes certain hazards. Understanding the dangers is critical for both patients and their families. Infection is one of the most prevalent CABG-related hazards. Despite strong cleanliness measures in hospitals, there is always the possibility of infection at the incision site or in the chest cavity. However, surgeons make great efforts to reduce this danger using sterilizing procedures and medicines.

Another typical concern is bleeding. CABG requires cutting into the chest cavity and manipulating blood arteries, thus there is a risk of severe bleeding during or after the operation.

Surgeons regularly monitor blood loss and take appropriate measures to limit it. Blood clots might also develop in the legs or lungs as a result of limited movement during the recuperation period. To avoid this, patients are often given blood thinners and advised to walk about as soon as possible following surgery.

Complications from anesthesia are also possible. Anesthesia is required to keep the patient asleep and pain-free throughout the treatment, although it may sometimes cause allergic responses or respiratory problems. However, anesthesiologists are highly trained experts who closely monitor the patient's vital signs during the procedure to guarantee their safety.

Finally, surgery may cause injury to nearby organs or tissues. Despite the accuracy of current surgical methods, the heart remains a fragile organ surrounded by essential tissues. Accidental harm to these structures is possible, although trained surgeons take all necessary precautions to reduce the risk.

Managing Complications During And Following Surgery

During CABG surgery, the surgical team is well-prepared for any difficulties that may occur. They have specialist equipment and pharmaceuticals on standby to treat conditions including bleeding, abnormal heartbeats, and low blood pressure. Surgeons are educated to make rapid judgments in high-pressure circumstances to achieve the best possible result for their patients.

Following surgery, patients are intensively watched in the intensive care unit (ICU) to discover and address any problems as early as possible. This involves monitoring vital signs, hydration balance, and blood oxygen levels. Nurses and physicians collaborate to guarantee patients' comfort and stability throughout the important post-operative time.

In certain situations, issues may not be discovered until after the patient has been released from the hospital. Infection, fluid accumulation around the heart, and graft failure are all common problems that might arise during the recovery period. Patients should keep an eye out for warning signals like fever, chest discomfort, or trouble breathing and seek medical assistance right once they appear.

Long-Term Risk And Preventive Measures

While CABG may successfully alleviate symptoms of coronary artery disease and enhance quality of life, it is crucial to note that some long-term hazards may remain. These include the formation of new blockages in bypass grafts, the advancement of underlying heart disease, and the necessity for future treatments.

To reduce these risks, patients are recommended to have a healthy lifestyle that includes frequent exercise, a balanced diet, and quitting smoking.

Statins, aspirin, and blood pressure drugs may also be administered to assist avoid future issues.

Regular follow-up meetings with a cardiologist are critical for tracking the patient's development and identifying any problems early on. These sessions usually involve physical examinations, imaging testing, and conversations regarding medication management. Patients who are proactive in their heart health may lower the risk of long-term problems and improve their quality of life after CABG surgery.

Importance Of Follow-Up Care

Follow-up treatment is critical to the long-term success of CABG surgery. It enables healthcare personnel to track the patient's recovery progress, evaluate the effectiveness of the bypass grafts, and make any required changes to their treatment plan. During follow-up sessions, patients should expect to have electrocardiograms (ECGs), echocardiograms, and stress tests performed to assess their heart function.

In addition to medical monitoring, follow-up treatment offers patients the chance to receive information and help in maintaining their cardiovascular health. This might include advice on medication adherence, dietary suggestions, and methods for lowering risk factors like high blood pressure or cholesterol.

Furthermore, follow-up treatment enables healthcare personnel to address patients' concerns or questions concerning their recovery or future prognosis. It is critical that patients feel educated and empowered enough to participate actively in their treatment.

Overall, consistent follow-up care is crucial for maximizing CABG surgical results and assisting patients in achieving the highest quality of life. Patients who interact with their healthcare team and follow their suggestions may benefit from better heart function and a lower risk of future issues.

CHAPTER 8

Lifestyle Changes And Long-Term Management

Dietary Tips For Heart Health

Diet is essential for preserving heart health, particularly after coronary artery bypass grafting (CABG). High cholesterol, high blood pressure, and obesity are all risk factors for heart disease, therefore your diet should prioritize lowering these. A diet high in fruits, vegetables, whole grains, lean meats, and healthy fats may greatly improve your cardiovascular health.

Fruit and Vegetable

Including a variety of colored fruits and vegetables in your diet gives important vitamins, minerals, and antioxidants. These nutrients assist in decreasing inflammation, regulate blood pressure, and promote overall heart health. Try to fill half of your plate with fruits and veggies at each meal.

Whole Grains

Whole grains such as brown rice, whole wheat bread, oats, and quinoa are high in fiber, which helps to decrease cholesterol and maintain a healthy weight. Choose whole grains over processed grains to improve your heart health.

Lean proteins

Choose lean protein sources such as chicken, fish, beans, lentils, and tofu. These protein sources include less saturated fat than red meats and processed meats, which may elevate cholesterol levels and increase the risk of heart disease.

Healthy fats

Incorporate healthy fats into your diet, such as olive oil, avocado, almonds, and seeds. These fats aid in lowering inflammation and improve cholesterol levels.

Moderation is essential, however, since all fats are high in calories.

Limit saturated and trans fats

Reduce your consumption of saturated fats from fatty meats, full-fat dairy products, and fried meals. Avoid trans fats contained in processed and packaged foods, which may boost bad cholesterol and increase the risk of heart disease.

Sodium Reduction

Limiting salt consumption is critical for controlling blood pressure and lowering the risk of cardiovascular disease. Choose fresh, natural meals over processed and packaged foods, which are often rich in salt. Instead of using salt, flavor your foods using herbs, spices, and lemon juice.

Maintain hydration by drinking lots of water throughout the day. Limit sugary drinks and instead drink water, herbal tea, or sparkling water with a dash of citrus for taste.

Exercise And Physical Activity Guidelines

Regular physical exercise is vital for preserving heart health and general well-being, particularly after CABG surgery. Exercise helps to strengthen the heart muscle, enhance circulation, decrease blood pressure, and control weight.

Aerobic exercise

Participate in moderate-intensity aerobic activities such as brisk walking, cycling, swimming, or dancing for at least 150 minutes each week, or 30 minutes on most days of the week. As your fitness level increases, progressively increase the time and intensity of your exercises.

Strength Training

Incorporate strength training workouts into your program at least twice a week. Concentrate on larger muscular groups such as the chest, back, legs, and arms. Strength exercise promotes muscle growth, boosts metabolism, and increases overall strength and endurance.

Flexibility and Balance

Incorporate flexibility and balance activities like yoga, tai chi, or stretching routines to increase joint mobility, decrease stiffness, and avoid falls. These exercises can help to relax and lower stress levels.

Pay attention to your body's response to exercise and change your intensity appropriately. If you develop chest discomfort, dizziness, or shortness of breath, stop exercising right away and get medical treatment.

Medications And Their Role In Recovery

Medications are essential for treating numerous risk factors and encouraging healing after CABG surgery. Your doctor may recommend a combination of drugs to reduce blood pressure, decrease cholesterol, avoid blood clots, and treat other underlying medical disorders.

Anti-platelet agents

Antiplatelet drugs like aspirin and clopidogrel help prevent blood clots from developing in the arteries, lowering the risk of a heart attack or stroke. Take these drugs exactly as directed, and share any concerns or adverse effects with your doctor.

Statins

Statins are cholesterol-lowering drugs that help decrease LDL (bad) cholesterol and lessen the risk of cardiovascular disease. These drugs may be administered to people who have high cholesterol or a history of heart disease.

Beta-Blockers

Beta-blockers lower heart rate and blood pressure, putting less strain on the heart and enhancing overall cardiac function. These drugs are often given to patients after CABG surgery to avoid angina, heart failure, and arrhythmias.

ACE inhibitors or ARBs

ACE inhibitors and angiotensin II receptor blockers (ARBs) work to relax blood arteries, reduce blood pressure, and enhance heart function. These drugs are often provided to people with heart failure or hypertension to lower the risk of future cardiovascular events.

Other medications

Other medicines, such as diuretics, calcium channel blockers, or antiarrhythmic agents, may be recommended to treat particular symptoms or illnesses.

Stress Management And Mental Health

Stress management and mental health are important factors in general well-being and cardiovascular health. Chronic stress may contribute to the development and progression of heart disease, thus it is important to discover good stress management strategies and prioritize mental health.

Relaxation techniques
Deep breathing, meditation, yoga, and progressive muscle relaxation are all relaxation practices that may help you decrease stress and develop a feeling of peace

and well-being. Incorporate these techniques into your routine to help you handle stress better.

Physical activity

Regular physical exercise not only benefits your physical health but also reduces stress and improves your mood. Engage in enjoyable activities, such as walking, swimming, dancing, or gardening, to increase endorphins and reduce stress.

Social Support

Maintaining strong social ties and seeking aid from friends, family, or support groups may help alleviate feelings of isolation and loneliness, both of which are risk factors for heart disease and poor mental health. Reach out to loved ones and connect with people who have gone through similar circumstances to provide and receive support.

Healthy coping strategies

Create effective coping methods for dealing with life's obstacles and failures. Instead of engaging in harmful behaviors such as smoking, excessive drinking, or overeating, seek alternate methods to deal with stress, such as writing, creative pursuits, or spending time in nature.

Professional Help

If you're having trouble coping with stress or have signs of anxiety or depression, don't be afraid to seek professional assistance from a therapist, counselor, or mental health professional. Talking to a skilled expert may offer you essential support and direction as you manage your mental health and well-being.

By applying these lifestyle adjustments and long-term management techniques, you may improve your recovery and lower your risk of future cardiovascular problems after coronary artery bypass grafting.

CHAPTER 9

Advancements And Alternatives In CABG

Latest Technological Advances In CABG

In recent years, coronary artery bypass grafting (CABG) technology has advanced significantly, resulting in better results and lower risks for individuals having the treatment. One major innovation is the development of less invasive methods like robotic-assisted CABG and endoscopic vein harvesting. In comparison to conventional open-heart surgery, these techniques allow for smaller incisions, less stress to surrounding tissues, and quicker recovery periods.

Another notable breakthrough is the use of sophisticated imaging methods such as intraoperative angiography and echocardiography.

These technologies enable surgeons to see the coronary arteries and heart structures more clearly throughout the surgery, allowing for more accurate transplant placement and optimum blood flow to the heart.

Furthermore, the introduction of new surgical equipment and technologies, such as high-definition cameras and robotic surgical systems, has improved the accuracy and efficacy of CABG treatments. These technologies allow surgeons to conduct complicated techniques with more precision and control, resulting in better surgical results and higher patient satisfaction.

Furthermore, the use of computer-assisted planning and navigation systems has transformed the planning and execution of CABG operations. These tools enable surgeons to preoperatively map the patient's coronary architecture, identify ideal transplant locations, and plan the surgical approach with unparalleled accuracy.

During the surgery, real-time navigation systems give visual feedback to guide the surgeon's motions, assuring accurate graft placement and reducing the possibility of mistakes.

Overall, technological developments have altered the area of CABG surgery, making it safer, more successful, and less intrusive for patients. As technology advances, further advancements are likely to improve the results of CABG and the lives of patients with coronary artery disease.

Alternative Surgical Techniques And Innovation

Aside from classic CABG surgery, various other surgical procedures and improvements have arisen in recent years, providing additional choices for patients with coronary artery disease. Off-pump CABG, often known as beating heart surgery, is a procedure for bypassing blocked coronary arteries that does not use a heart-lung bypass machine.

Instead, the heart beats during the treatment, enabling the surgeon to graft the bypasses onto the moving heart tissue. Off-pump CABG is linked with lower risks of complications including stroke and kidney damage, and it may be preferable for certain patients, especially those with pre-existing diseases that increase the risk of problems from traditional CABG.

Another option is hybrid CABG, which combines standard surgical revascularization and percutaneous coronary intervention (PCI). In hybrid CABG, the surgeon performs CABG to bypass severely obstructed coronary arteries, whilst PCI is utilized to treat less severe blockages or residual disease in other coronary vessels. This hybrid method enables a personalized treatment plan that targets each patient's particular requirements, possibly increasing results and lowering the need for further treatments.

Furthermore, advances in grafting materials have broadened the alternatives for CABG surgery. In addition to typical vein transplants taken from the patient's leg or arm, surgeons may now use arterial grafts such as the internal mammary artery and radial artery. Arterial grafts are known to have better long-term patency rates than vein grafts and may be preferable, especially in younger patients or those with diabetes.

Additionally, tissue engineering and regenerative medicine technologies show promise for the future of CABG surgery. Researchers are looking for ways to build new blood arteries or restore damaged heart tissue using stem cells or other biological agents. These techniques have the potential to increase the success rate of CABG surgeries and the long-term results for patients with coronary artery disease.

A Comparison Of CABG With Other Treatments (Angioplasty, Stenting)

When contemplating treatment choices for coronary artery disease, patients and healthcare professionals must compare the advantages and dangers of CABG against other alternatives such as angioplasty and stent placement. Angioplasty, also known as percutaneous coronary intervention (PCI), is a procedure that involves inflating a balloon within a constricted coronary artery to enlarge it and restore blood flow. Stenting, a typical follow-up to angioplasty, involves inserting a thin mesh tube (stent) into the artery to keep it open.

One benefit of angioplasty and stenting is that they are less intrusive than CABG surgery, with shorter hospital stays and quicker recovery periods. Furthermore, these treatments may often be conducted under local anesthetic and conscious sedation, eliminating the requirement for general anesthesia and its accompanying hazards.

However, CABG may be chosen in certain circumstances, especially for individuals with complicated coronary artery disease with numerous blockages. CABG allows for more comprehensive revascularization by bypassing blocked arteries with grafts, while angioplasty and stenting may only address the local region of blockage. In certain patient groups, CABG is linked with fewer repeat treatments and greater long-term survival than angioplasty and stenting.

Furthermore, CABG may be the preferable choice for patients with diabetes or left main coronary artery disease, since it has been found to provide better results than angioplasty and stenting in these high-risk categories. Furthermore, CABG may be suggested for individuals with significant coronary artery disease who are not candidates for angioplasty and stenting owing to anatomical or technological limitations.

Finally, the decision between CABG and alternative therapies is based on several considerations, including the patient's general health, the amount and complexity of coronary artery disease, and personal preferences. A detailed conversation between the patient and their healthcare professional is required to find the best treatment method for each unique instance.

Future Trends In Coronary Artery Surgery

Looking forward, numerous intriguing innovations in coronary artery surgery promise to enhance patient outcomes and quality of treatment. One new trend is the use of minimally invasive and robotic-assisted procedures for CABG, which allow for even smaller incisions, less stress, and shorter recovery periods than existing methods. These developments may broaden the eligibility for CABG to a wider group of patients, lowering the total burden of coronary artery disease.

Furthermore, developments in imaging technology and intraoperative navigation devices are projected to continue, allowing surgeons to execute CABG procedures with remarkable precision and accuracy. Real-time imaging and guiding systems will enable optimum graft placement and assure the long-term patency of bypass grafts, resulting in better results and fewer postoperative problems.

Furthermore, customized medicine methods are expected to play a larger role in the future of coronary artery surgery. Healthcare practitioners may improve results and reduce the risk of problems after CABG by adapting treatment regimens to specific patient variables like as genetics, comorbidities, and lifestyle. This tailored approach may include sophisticated biomarkers, genetic testing, and predictive analytics to help guide treatment choices and enhance patient care.

Furthermore, continuing research in tissue engineering and regenerative medicine shows promise in the creation of innovative medicines to improve cardiac regeneration and stimulate vascular expansion. These novel techniques might transform the management of coronary artery disease by offering new options for restoring blood flow to the ischemic heart and improving cardiac function in individuals with advanced illness.

To summarize, the future of coronary artery surgery seems promising, with continuing advances in technology, surgical methods, and customized medicine projected to enhance patient outcomes and quality of care. By embracing these developments and remaining at the forefront of research and development, cardiac surgeons may continue to make substantial advances in the treatment of coronary artery disease, improving the lives of patients all around the globe.

CHAPTER 10

Patient Stories And Testimonials

Challenges Faced During Recovery

Recovery after coronary artery bypass grafting (CABG) surgery may be difficult, both physically and emotionally. Many patients face a variety of challenges while they recover and regain their strength after surgery. One prevalent issue is pain management. Following the treatment, patients may feel discomfort or soreness at the incision sites or in the chest. This pain might make it difficult to move around or do everyday tasks, resulting in irritation and exhaustion. However, healthcare experts usually prescribe pain relievers to assist ease these symptoms and enhance the patient's comfort throughout recuperation.

Another barrier during rehabilitation is adapting to new lifestyle habits. Following CABG surgery, individuals often need to make considerable changes to their diet, exercise regimen, and general lifestyle to improve heart health and avoid subsequent issues. This transition phase might be difficult for some patients, particularly those who were not used to good behaviors before surgery. However, with the help of healthcare experts, family members, and support groups, patients may gradually adjust to these changes and adopt a heart-healthy lifestyle for long-term well-being.

Additionally, some patients may have emotional difficulties throughout the rehabilitation phase. It is fairly unusual for people to experience anxiety, depression, or overwhelm after a major operation like CABG. These sentiments may be caused by anxiety about their health, dread of problems, or uncertainty about the future. Patients must acknowledge and treat these feelings, whether via therapy, support groups, or just chatting freely with family members. Patients who acknowledge and process their emotions may better deal with the emotional aspects of recovery and concentrate on their overall healing journey.

Furthermore, problems like as infection or fluid accumulation might develop throughout the recuperation phase, complicating the patient's trip. Infections at the surgical site or in the chest cavity might delay healing and need extra medical treatments, such as antibiotics or drainage operations. Similarly, fluid collection around the heart or lungs may cause breathing problems and pain, demanding immediate medical intervention to avoid consequences.

Despite these obstacles, many patients discover strength and resilience as they recover after CABG surgery. Individuals may overcome hurdles and achieve success with tenacity, patience, and the assistance of healthcare practitioners and loved ones. Each patient's journey is unique, but by sharing their stories and learning from others who have been down a similar road, people may face the obstacles of recovery with bravery and resolve.

Tips And Advice From Others Who Have Had The Procedure

Patients who have had coronary artery bypass grafting (CABG) surgery often have useful insights and tips to share with those going through a similar experience. Their own experiences may provide comfort, wisdom, and encouragement to those preparing for or recuperating from the treatment. Here are some ideas and guidance from folks who have been through CABG:

1. **Follow your doctor's orders:** One of the most crucial pieces of advice for CABG patients is to rigorously follow the suggestions and directions given by your healthcare team. This involves taking prescribed drugs, going to follow-up visits, and following food and lifestyle advice.

You may improve your recovery and lower your risk of problems by carefully following your doctor's directions.

2. Listen to your body: During the rehabilitation process, it's critical to pay attention to any warning signals or symptoms. If you have unexpected chest discomfort, shortness of breath, dizziness, or other serious symptoms, get medical assistance immediately. Ignoring symptoms might cause treatment delays and consequences.

3. Take it slowly: Recovery following CABG surgery is a long process that demands patience and endurance. It's critical not to push yourself too hard or try to resume regular activities too soon. Allow your body enough time to mend and rebuild strength at its own pace. Begin with easy exercises such as walking and gradually increase the intensity as recommended by your healthcare provider.

4. **Concentrate on self-care:** Self-care is critical throughout the recovery time to encourage healing and general well-being. This includes getting enough sleep, eating a healthy diet, reducing stress, and using relaxation methods like deep breathing or meditation. Prioritize self-care activities that will feed your body, mind, and soul.

5. **Seek help:** Don't be afraid to ask for help from family members, friends, or support groups throughout your recovery process. A robust support network may provide emotional encouragement, practical aid, and friendship when faced with hardship. Share your problems, anxieties, and achievements with trustworthy people who can provide empathy and understanding.

6. Maintaining a good attitude may have a big impact on your recovery process. While it is common to have ups and downs along the road, try to concentrate on the progress you've made and the milestones you've met.

Celebrate modest triumphs while being optimistic about the future. Maintaining a positive outlook might help you remain motivated and resilient throughout the rehabilitation process.

Overall, CABG patients' advice and ideas highlight the value of patience, self-care, and support during the recovery process. By implementing these tactics into your recovery plan and gaining inspiration from individuals who have overcome similar obstacles, you may maximize your recovery and move on with confidence and hope.

Overcoming Heart Disease

Overcoming heart disease is a process that needs dedication, endurance, and support from healthcare providers, family members, and the community. Individuals diagnosed with coronary artery disease (CAD) or other types of heart disease must make proactive efforts to control the illness and enhance their heart health.

Adopting a heart-healthy lifestyle is one of the most effective ways to overcome heart disease. This involves changing your diet to eat less saturated fat, cholesterol, and salt while eating more fruits, vegetables, healthy grains, and lean meats. Regular physical exercise is also important for building heart muscle, boosting circulation, and lowering the risk of cardiovascular disease. Aim to do at least 150 minutes of moderate-intensity activity each week, such as brisk walking, cycling, or swimming.

In addition to diet and exercise, treating risk factors such as high blood pressure, high cholesterol, diabetes, and obesity is critical for avoiding the advancement of cardiovascular disease. This may include following your doctor's recommended medicines, checking blood sugar levels, keeping a healthy weight, and, if you smoke, stopping. Addressing these risk factors may dramatically lower the chance of heart-related problems while also improving overall heart health.

Individuals with extensive coronary artery disease or who have had heart attacks may benefit from coronary artery bypass grafting (CABG) surgery to restore blood flow to the heart and relieve symptoms. While CABG surgery is a serious treatment, it may save many patients' lives and allow them to return to a full and active lifestyle.

Furthermore, mental well-being is critical to conquering cardiac disease. Living with a chronic ailment may be difficult, both physically and emotionally, thus it is important to address the psychosocial elements of cardiac disease. Seek help from mental health specialists, attend support groups, and rely on family and friends for emotional support during stressful times. Deep breathing, meditation, and mindfulness are all stress-management practices that may help you relax and decrease anxiety.

Overall, conquering heart disease requires a multifaceted strategy that considers physical, mental, and behavioral issues.

Individuals with heart disease may empower themselves to live well and decrease the risk of problems by taking proactive actions to manage the illness, adopting a heart-healthy lifestyle, and seeking help when required. Remember that you are not alone on this path, and there are tools and assistance available to help you overcome obstacles and live despite heart disease.

Conclusion

Finally, the voyage of learning Coronary Artery Bypass Grafting (CABG) offers a diverse approach to coronary artery disease (CAD). CABG is a cornerstone in the care of CAD, providing patients with the opportunity to enhance their quality of life and live longer.

First, studying the anatomy and pathophysiology of CAD gives the framework for understanding why CABG is required. CAD, which is defined as the accumulation of plaque in the coronary arteries, reduces blood flow to the heart muscle, causing symptoms such as chest discomfort and shortness of breath. Understanding this disease process emphasizes the need for therapies like CABG to restore proper blood circulation to the heart.

CABG surgery includes rerouting blood flow around blocked or constricted coronary arteries using grafts obtained from other regions of the body, most often the saphenous vein or internal mammary artery. Cardiac surgeons may successfully bypass clogged arteries, restoring blood flow to ischemic heart tissue, thanks to their rigorous surgical expertise and technological technology.

Furthermore, studying the indications and contraindications for CABG clarifies the patient selection procedure. While CABG is a very beneficial therapy for many patients with CAD, it may not be appropriate for everyone. The level and location of coronary artery disease, general health state, and patient preferences are all important considerations when deciding whether to have CABG surgery.

Postoperative care and rehabilitation are essential parts of the CABG experience. Close monitoring during the initial postoperative period aids in the identification and management of any problems such as bleeding, infection, or arrhythmias. Furthermore, organized rehabilitation programs help with recovery, increase cardiovascular fitness, and encourage long-term adherence to lifestyle changes that reduce the risk of future cardiac episodes.

Looking beyond the technical elements, it is critical to acknowledge CABG's enormous influence on patients' lives. For many people, CABG is not merely a medical procedure, but also a transforming event that provides hope and the possibility of a fresh lease on life. CABG may improve patients' overall well-being and quality of life by reducing symptoms and restoring functional ability.

To summarize, the comprehensive guide to understanding Coronary Artery Bypass Grafting covers not only the surgical method but also the larger context of CAD therapy, patient selection, and postoperative care. CABG continues to play an important role in fighting coronary artery disease and improving outcomes for countless people throughout the globe because of a holistic strategy that combines medical knowledge, surgical competence, and compassionate patient care.

THE END